Fishes for Danierr:
Over 100 seafood recipes

Niko Novakovic

Alabama Shrimp Bake 1 cup melted butter or margarine 3/4 cup lemon juice 3/4 cup Worcestershire sauce 1 tablespoon salt 1 tablespoon coarsely ground pepper 1 teaspoon dried rosemary 1/8 teaspoon ground red pepper 1 tablespoon hot sauce 3 minced garlic cloves 2 1/2 pounds unpeeled large or jumbo shrimp 2 lemons, thinly sliced Fresh rosemary sprigs put away.

Use ice water to wash the shrimp; well, drain. In an ungreased 13 x 9 x 2-inch baking dish, layer the shrimp, lemon slices, and onion slices. Over the shrimp, spread the butter mixture. Cover and bake at 400 degrees F for 20 to 25 minutes, basting occasionally with pan juices, until shrimp are pink. Decorate with new

rosemary branches.

6 servings

1 pound extra-large shrimp, peeled and deveined, tails remaining on 1/2 cup all-purpose flour Vegetable oil Combine eggs, milk, salt, and pepper in a shallow bowl. Alabama Shrimp Bake 3 Almost

Shrimp Paesano Shrimp Dip the shrimp in the mixture, then lightly coat them with flour.

In a sauté pan, heat the oil until it is hot, then add four to six shrimp at a time, giving them plenty of room to cook. It's vital that shrimp are not close to one another or contact.) After browning one side, flip them over and brown the other side. Bake on a baking sheet in an oven preheated to 350 degrees Fahrenheit or cook until done. Make the sauce in the meantime.

Sauce: 1 1/2 cups (3 sticks) cold butter cut into 1-inch pieces; 1 medium lemon juice; 1 minced clove of garlic; 2 tablespoons minced fresh parsley. In a large saucepan, combine the butter, lemon juice, and garlic. Whisk the mixture constantly over medium-low heat until the butter is just melted and thickened. Mix in parsley, then eliminate from heat.

Placing cooked shrimp on top of pool sauce The leftover sauce goes well with seafood that has been grilled or broiled.)

Serves 3-4 people

Nearly Shrimp Paesano 4

Amaretto Shrimp

Yields 4 to 5 servings

1/2 cup spread

1/3 cup amaretto

1/3 cup cut almonds

2 teaspoons granulated sugar

1/2 teaspoon ground cinnamon

1/8 teaspoon cayenne pepper

1 pound huge shrimp, stripped and deveined, tails left on

In a huge skillet, dissolve the spread over medium intensity.

Stir in the sugar, cinnamon, cayenne pepper, amaretto, and almonds until the sugar is dissolved. Add the shrimp and cook until just pink, 3 to 5 minutes.

Serve right away with hot rice.

 Amaretto Shrimp, 5 Avocado Crepes with Crab, 1 Large Avocado, 6 Eggs, 3/4 Cup of Flour, Salt, and Pepper, 3/4 Cup of Milk, 3/4 Cup of Water, Butter, 3 Cups of Cream Sauce, 1/3 Cup of Diced Gruyere Cheese, 1 Tablespoon Worcestershire Sauce, 1 1/2

Cans of Crab Meat, 1/2 Cup of Grated Cheese, Mash Avocado; Add the flour, salt, and eggs. Beat until smooth and continuously mix in milk and water.

Melt 1/3 teaspoon of butter in a 6-inch pan over high heat. Pour in 4 tablespoons avocado hitter. Brown the pancake by tilting the pan to cover the bottom. Cook the other side by turning. Use up all of the batter.

Sauce, heat Cook until the sauce thickens by adding the

Gruyere cheese. Take off the heat. Add

Worcestershire sauce. Mix in the crabmeat.

Roll each pancake up and add a small amount of the filling. In a large shallow baking dish coated with butter, arrange the pancakes in a single layer. Sprinkle with cheese grates. Butter the spots. Bake the cheese at 425°F until it melts.

Serves 6-8 people

Avocado Crepes with Crab 6 Backyard Shrimp Fest 1/2 cup Old Bay seasoning, 2 tablespoons salt, 4 quarts water, 1 (12-ounce) can beer (optional) 8 medium red potatoes, cut in half, 2 large sweet onions, cut in wedges, 2 pounds lean smoked sausage, cut in 2 inch lengths, 8 ears fresh corn, cut in half, and 4 pounds large shrimp in shells Add the onions and potatoes; cook for eight minutes over high heat.

Add smoked sausage to the onions, potatoes, and keep on cooking on high for 5 minutes. Toss in the corn;

keep on bubbling for 7 minutes. Add the shelled shrimp; cook for 4 minutes.

Remove the cooking liquid. Empty items in pot into a few enormous dishes, shallow buckets or hill on a

paper–covered outdoor table. If you like, you can add more seasoning.

Serves eight large portions Serving Tip: Use paper plates and newsprint to cover the picnic or patio table to cut down on cleanup. Mound the tents on top of the paper after removing the water from the pot. Gather the group around the table and have a good time peeling and eating the shrimp. For the shrimp shells, provide bowls or pails that are empty.

Lawn Shrimp Fest 7

Heated Shellfish with Bleu Cheddar

1/2 pound stripped youthful potatoes

4 tablespoons milk

4 tablespoons olive oil

2 tablespoons slashed flat-leaf parsley

2 dozen stout, new shellfish

Salt and pepper, to taste

2 egg yolks

4 tablespoon dry white wine

2/3 cup cream

3 ounces disintegrated bleu cheddar

Cook the potatoes in salted, bubbling water until delicate. Use a fork to combine the milk, olive oil, and parsley into a smooth mash.

Remove the bodies from the oysters' shells after they have been opened, preserve the juice, and set them aside. Remove the top shell and thoroughly clean the bottom shell.

In a double boiler, combine the egg yolks and wine, beating constantly throughout, and cook until the mixture doubles in volume.

Combine the Bleu cheese and the cream in a different pan. After two to three minutes at a boil, turn off the heat. Gently incorporate the oyster juice into the egg yolks after adding it.

Mash the potatoes in the oyster shells before serving. Cover the oysters with the sauce before placing them on top. They should be cooked for five minutes under the grill to produce a golden brown mixture.

Serve warm.

Baked Oysters with Bleu Cheese 8 Baked Scallops with Garlic Sauce 1 and a half pounds of bay scallops, cut in half, 3 cloves of garlic, mashed, 1/4 cup (1/2 stick) margarine, melted, 10 firm white mushrooms, sliced Light dash of onion salt, dash of freshly grated pepper, 1/3 cup seasoned bread crumbs, 1 teaspoon finely minced fresh parsley, and a damp paper towel. Squash garlic cloves and add to margarine; mix well to mix.

Stay warm. In the bottom of a baking dish, put a little of the melted garlic sauce; add the

mushrooms and season. Put the scallops on top of the mushrooms. The remaining garlic sauce can be drizzled over scallops. Reserve one tablespoon. Sprinkle with parsley, bread crumbs, and the remaining garlic sauce. Bake at 375 degrees Fahrenheit, preheated, until the top is nicely browned and hot.

Heated Scallops with Garlic Sauce 9

Heated Stuffed Shrimp

24 enormous shrimp

1 medium onion, minced

1 green pepper, slashed

6 tablespoons margarine, separated

1 cup new crab meat or 1 (7 1/2 ounce) can

1 teaspoon dry mustard

Paprika

1 teaspoon Worcestershire sauce

1/2 teaspoon salt

2 tablespoons mayonnaise

2 tablespoons flour

1 cup milk

1 tablespoon sherry wine, or more

Ground Parmesan cheddar

Clean and eliminate heads and shells from shrimp, leaving tails. Part shrimp and open level. In 4 tablespoons of the butter, sauté the pepper and onion until soft but not browned. Add the crab meat, dry mustard,

Worcestershire sauce, salt and mayonnaise. Place aside.

Utilizing the remaining two tablespoons of butter, flour, and milk, make a white sauce. Add the sherry to the mixture of crab meat. Blend well; stuff the butterflied shrimp with the crab meat and dab with extra margarine. Paprika and Parmesan cheese are lightly sprinkled on top. Place everything in a shallow baking pan and bake for 25 to 30 minutes at 350 degrees F.

Serves 4-6 people.

10 Baked Stuffed Shrimp 10 large shrimp 1 1/2 sleeves Ritz crackers, crushed 1/2 pound butter, melted 1 tablespoon horseradish 1 tablespoon Worcestershire sauce 1 tablespoon Tabasco sauce 1 teaspoon garlic salt Lemon Shell and devein the shrimp. Put

shrimp on a cookie sheet that has been greased. Crushed crackers, butter, horseradish, Tabasco, Worcestershire, and garlic salt are mixed in. Stuff the shrimp with it. Bake for 15 minutes at 400 degrees Fahrenheit.

Present with lemon wedges.

Heated Stuffed Shrimp 11

Heated Stuffed Shrimp

25 to 30 enormous shrimp

3/4 stick (6 tablespoons) spread or margarine

6 ribs celery, slashed

1 enormous onion, slashed

3 cove leaves

1 bundle green onions, slashed

1 bundle new parsley, slashed

1 pound crabmeat (knot or paw)

Salt, dark and red peppers, to taste

Around 3/4 of a medium-size French bread portion

1 cup prepared bread morsels

Strip crude shrimp, leaving tail segment on shrimp. Butterfly and devein shrimp. Keep in the fridge until you make the dressing.

Sauté the celery, onions, and bay leaves in butter or margarine in a medium skillet until tender. Add parsley and green onions. Sauté until soft. Obtain the bay leaves.

French bread should be punctured. After soaking the bread in cold water, squeeze out the majority of the water. Using your hands, cut the bread into small pieces and place them in a mixing bowl. Bread should have a mixture of parsley, celery, and onions. Add salt and pepper to the crabmeat.

Wrap some of the dressing around the shrimp by hand, leaving the tail exposed, and serve. Over the stuffing, roll or sprinkle seasoned bread crumbs. Put on daintily lubed treat sheet.

Bake for about 30 minutes at 350 degrees Fahrenheit.

25 to 30 stuffed shrimp are produced.

Baltimore Crab Cakes

1 pound. 1 large, beaten egg 1/4 cup mayonnaise or salad dressing 2 tablespoons finely chopped scallions 1/4 teaspoon garlic salt 1/8 teaspoon white pepper 2 teaspoons dried onion flakes 3/4 teaspoon dried parsley flakes 1 cup all-purpose flour 1/4 cup melted butter or margarine Combine the first 11 ingredients; shape into 6 patties. Use flour to coat; chill somewhere around 60 minutes.

The patties should be cooked for four minutes on each side, or until golden, in butter, in a skillet over medium heat.

13 barbecued oysters from Baltimore: 3 cups oysters, 3/4 cup flour, salt and pepper to taste, and 1 1/2 cups barbecue sauce. Blend flour, salt and pepper in earthy colored basic food item pack. Shake shellfish in flour combination.

In hot oil, sauté oysters just long enough to form a crust, but not long enough to cook them through. Cover the oysters with barbecue sauce in a rectangular baking dish. Bake for 20 to 25 minutes at 350 degrees Fahrenheit.

Barbecued Oysters 14

Barbecue Shrimp 2 smashed garlic cloves 2 bay leaves 6 pounds fresh Gulf shrimp, 20 to 25 per pound, 1/4 cup lemon juice 1/2 pound salted butter 1/2 pound margarine 2 teaspoons paprika 1 newly purchased 4 ounce can black pepper Preheat the oven to 300 degrees Fahrenheit. Scrub the inside of one or two baking pans large enough to hold all the shrimp with the garlic cloves.

To get as much garlic oil as possible in there, squeeze it in.

The garlic itself should be thrown away, but you should keep the stray specks. Put two bay leaves at the pan's bottom.

The shrimp should be washed and patted dry before being placed in the baking pan on their sides, crowded together and slightly overlapped. Lemon juice should be used to cover the shrimp.

Distribute the cubes of butter and margarine over the shrimp. Apply the paprika to it. Sprinkle enough black pepper over the shrimp to create a layer of black that can be felt. Miss no spots! (Also, you don't need to utilize the entire can, by the same token.)

For 15 minutes, bake the shrimp in an oven preheated to 300 degrees F. Make sure they are finished; You are there when the meat separates from the shells. Soft, wrinkly shells are not what you want. If necessary, return the shrimp to the oven for a short time.

The shrimp should be served on soup plates with a lot of sauce and toasted French bread.

Additionally, plenty of bibs and perhaps napkins.

15 Barbecued Shrimp 5 pounds of shrimp with heads Salt and pepper to taste 3 bay leaves 1/4 cup of oregano 1/3 bottle of garlic juice 1 teaspoon Tabasco® sauce 2 pounds of butter 6 large or 8 small lemons Arrange the shrimp in an even layer in a large casserole or metal pan. Salt and pepper them completely until you think they are gone. Disintegrate cove leaves and sprinkle equitably over shrimp. Sprinkle oregano, garlic

juice and Tabasco over shrimp.

Melt butter in a separate pan. Butter should be infused with lemon juice, pulp, and seeds. Pour the mixture over the shrimp. Bake for 30 to 40 minutes, covered, at 350 degrees Fahrenheit.

Serves 6 to 8 people.

 Grilled Shrimp 16

 Grilled Shrimp

2 pounds new, unpeeled shrimp

4 stems celery with leaves, diced

1/2 teaspoon garlic powder

3 lemons, cut into wedges

2 tablespoon broke dark pepper

3/4 cup spread or margarine, cut into 3D shapes

Lemon wedges (for embellish)

2 tablespoons Worcestershire sauce

2 tablespoons salt

3/4 teaspoon hot sauce

Wash shrimp completely and place in a huge shallow dish. Include garlic and celery. Apply lemon juice to the top. Sprinkle the shrimp with the remaining ingredients, excluding the lemon wedges, and dot with butter.

Under the broiler, repeatedly stir the shrimp until the butter melts and the shrimp begin to turn pink (about 5 minutes). Reduce the temperature to 350 degrees Fahrenheit and bake for an additional 20 minutes, stirring frequently, until the shrimp are cooked through. Shrimp will become mushy if they are overcooked. Check for completion.

Use lemon wedges as a garnish.

Flavor improves on the off chance that shrimp are cooked somewhat early and, warmed, however don't overcook.

 Barbecued Shrimp: 17 Basic Shrimp: 2 quarts heavily salted water; 2 bay leaves; 5 whole cloves of garlic; 1 large celery rib coarsely chopped; 1 halved clove of garlic; Tabasco® sauce; 1 pinch each of thyme and basil; Heat to the point of boiling, then, at that point, switch off the

heat. Bright pink shrimp indicate readiness.

Basic Shrimp 18 Batter-Fried Shrimp 2 eggs, 1/2 cup milk, 1 cup all-purpose flour, mixed before measuring, 1 teaspoon baking powder, 1 teaspoon salt, 2 teaspoons vegetable oil, 2 pounds fresh or frozen whole shrimp, oil (for deep-fat frying), and a choice of sauces (following) Beat the eggs and milk together until they form a frothy mixture. Flour, baking powder, and salt, sift together. Include in egg mixture; Beat in the oil until the mixture is well-blended and smooth. Place aside.

Remove the shrimp's tails from their shells. Under running, cold water, remove the shrimp's shells if they are frozen. Cut along the outside curve about halfway through. Remove the vein; wash shrimp and smooth so

they stay open. Use paper towels to drain well.

In a deep-fat fryer or kettle, add enough oil or shortening to cover the shrimp and heat to 375 degrees Fahrenheit. Dip each shrimp in the batter and fry for about 4 minutes, or until golden brown and puffy. Use paper towels to drain.

Serve promptly with selection of sauces.

Orange Sauce 1 cup Smucker's Sweet Orange Marmalade 1 clove of garlic 1 whole ginger root or 1/2 teaspoon ground ginger Combine all of the ingredients in a saucepan and cook, stirring constantly, over low heat until the mixture bubbles. Ginger and garlic should be removed.

approximately 1 cup.

Grape–Horseradish Sauce

1 cup Smucker's Grape Jam

1 tablespoon arranged horseradish

1/4 cup catsup

Consolidate all fixings.

Plum Hot Sauce 1 cup Smucker's Plum Preserves 1 to 2 very finely minced garlic cloves 2 teaspoons soy sauce 1 teaspoon pepper In a saucepan, combine all of the ingredients and cook, stirring occasionally, for at least 5 minutes or until the garlic is cooked. Cool briefly after removing from the heat.

approximately 1 cup.

www.ingramcontent.com/pod-product-compliance
Lightning Source LLC
Chambersburg PA
CBHW051900250726
48659CB00006B/2313